Laughing Through A Second Pregnancy

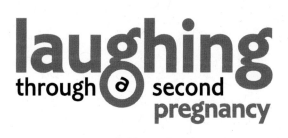

A Memoir
By Vanessa Shields

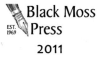

2011

© Vanessa Shields 2011

Library and Archives Canada Cataloguing in Publication

Shields, Vanessa, 1978-
    Laughing through a second pregnancy : a memoir
    / Vanessa Shields.

ISBN 978-0-88753-482-9

    1. Pregnancy--Humor. 2. Pregnancy--Popular works.
I. Title.

RG525.S55 2011   618.2'00207   C2010-907459-9

Black Moss Press is published at 2450 Byng Road, Windsor, Ontario, Canada N8W 3E8. Black Moss books are distributed in Canada and the U.S. by LitDisCo. All orders should be directed there.

Black Moss acknowledges the generous support for its publishing program from The Canada Council for the Arts and The Ontario Arts Council.

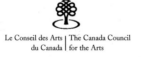

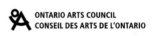

Printed in Canada

For my husband Nick
For our son Jett, our firstborn
For our daughter Miller, our second born

It's not luck, it's love…again

Table of Contents

Part One: Life Changes - Again

Happy Waddling	11
Obvious Forgettings	14
Your Child Is Perfect	16
The "What If" Questions	18
A Crappy Reality	21
Clean Purge Prepare	26
Second Baby Go-Aheads	29
Date Night	34

Part Two: Boobs

Mom Boobs	37
To Boob Or To Bottle?	39
Taste Test	42
Leaky Loo	44
Cold Turkey Boobs	46

Part Three: Vaginas 101

Changes To My Girl	53
A Girl And A Mirror	55
Scent Of A Woman	56
MacGyver Mom	59
The Practice Vagina	61

Kegels Shmegels	64
Between My Legs	66
Self Serve Or On The Side	68
Humping And Jumping	71

Part Four: Bittersweet Body Battles

Remembering Belly	77
You're An Eight	79
Fart Fests And Burp-a-thons	81
Baby Got Back Pain	84
If A Cramp Happens, Does Anybody Hear It?	86
Eighth Wonder	88
Bittersweet Body Battle	90
The Demon Woman	93
Leftovers	96

Part 5: Final Conceptions

The Cross It Off Tour	101
Spiritual Things	104
Neither Tom Nor Cruise	107
Tearing Off The Layers	109
Am Pregnant – Will Travel	112

Life Changes – Again

plans

I always planned on having children, two by the time I was thirty, then tie up my tubes and be a mom. Today, I'm twenty-seven, pregnant with the first child, fourteen weeks in me, and mentally preparing for the second. I take nausea with gusto as it collides with exhaustion.

Was I blessed with a glimpse, a fate without details that I stored in my heart to hold into reality? To feel into life?

Happy Waddling

No matter how naked it has made me feel to write this book, I've written it. I've endeavored to be frank, open, and without shame. I've written freely about vagina, fart-smell, sex, food, vagina, love, family, work, money and have I mentioned vagina?

The thing is, these subjects need writing. I've written them for my husband, for inquiring husbands and life partners, for those going it alone by choice or by circumstance and for you, dear reader. This stuff needs to be talked about because it is real, it is beautiful and it is miraculous. I too wanted to know. I wanted an inside story. I just couldn't find the book. So I wrote the book. If only I could have melted in some savoury chocolate for good measure.

This is not a "how to" book. It's a memoir, a record, a glimpse, a statement. It may not change the world, but it's real and true, and it wasn't my intention to change anyone or anything when I wrote it. It is what it is.

When I began writing this book, my forearms couldn't help but rest on the sides of my bulging belly. My t-shirt pulled tightly over new stretch marks. They were thicker. Stronger. There I was, once again, back in my belly – pregnant with life shifting all around me, within me. Waddling down a path I wasn't quite sure about. I knew what was going to happen at the end after hours of pain – I'd be holding a perfect child.

When I was pregnant with Jett, our firstborn, I didn't think I'd get to the point where I just wanted the baby to come out. I had loved being pregnant. I had loved the feeling of the baby moving around in my giant belly and watching its knee or elbow or heel slide beneath my skin. I had loved watching life growing inside of me. I had been naïve about how much it would hurt during labour.

The second time around, I knew how much it was going to hurt. I was scared. Scared that I had to go through labour again. It took twenty-seven hours to get Jett out of me and I was in pain or throwing up the whole time. I was afraid I'd have the same experience with baby number two. The heaviness and exhaustion were intense and started earlier in the pregnancy. You know that point you reach when all you want is to get the baby out? Well, I reached that point earlier during my second pregnancy, despite my growing dread of what was to come during labour.

Ultimately, for both pregnancies, it wasn't up to me when the baby came out. The baby decides when he's coming out and no one else. I am thankful that pregnancy lasts nine months because it takes that long to convince ourselves that we'll go through labour again!

The nine months of my first pregnancy were so much about *me,* and getting my self physically, emotionally and spiritually ready to be a mother. I asked myself hard questions like: Who am I? What do I believe in? What's the most important thing I want to teach my child? Am I eating too much chocolate? The second time I was pregnant I had different questions, but they were still important: Where am I? If there is a God, can she make my labour quick? What am I forgetting to teach my child?

The second nine months were about remembering how I did it the first time and quickly realizing that everything, from my body to my mind to my soul, was different. I still had the same answers to the tough questions. I'd been there, solidified that. I knew I was eating too much chocolate!

I did my best to make sure that the last days before Miller was born were peaceful. I gave myself the time and freedom to rest when I could, to eat what I wanted. This was a challenge considering I worked full-time until two days before Miller was born because my hubby Nick and I were making a feature film. I was running to the set and office, and taking care of Jett. Even during all this, I made time for *me*. It was sparse but it was there.

Everyone told me how much harder having two kids would be, and that my life would change drastically – again. I wasn't scared when they told me this. Generally, I knew what I was in for. I told myself that it would be totally doable. Twice the fun and the exhaustion.

Obvious Forgettings

I was thankful that my body remembered how to be pregnant again because my mind forgot pretty much everything. From what food I was supposed to eat to how to lie in bed, I couldn't remember anything. It was amazing to me that this happened because I promised myself that I wouldn't forget a thing. I cherished each moment while I was pregnant with Jett. I thought that the remembering would come back to my mind like the chub came back to my belly. That wasn't the case. As my body grew in size I remembered how physically taxing carrying a baby could be.

There was a mind-body connection that was undeniable when I was pregnant. I felt this connection during both pregnancies. But with Miller, my mind, in general, was busy with non-baby related things like work and raising Jett. I couldn't stop my life to bask in the experience of being pregnant.

I forgot how forgetful pregnancy made me. I forgot how clumsy I could get and how I could barely do dishes because I couldn't reach the sink with my big belly in the way. I forgot how challenging shaving and other general body maintenance was when my tummy was so huge. I forgot what it was like to have a period!

Since I nursed Miller for quite some time, I didn't get my period until about eighteen months after she was born. Including being pregnant, that meant I didn't have a period for over two years. I forgot what it was like to get cramps, zits, and PMS. I forgot about tampons too! Of course I knew I'd start getting my period again but I'd forgotten all the not-so-fun stuff that comes along with it.

Mostly, I forgot what to do with an infant. It may seem silly but it's the truth. I was so used to being with Jett who was talking and running all over the place that I forgot some obvious things. For example, infants need to be held – a lot. They can't sit up alone. They can't tell me what's wrong. They are small, and they need to be burped after every feeding or else they barf. I was baffled when I fed Miller and she fell asleep so peacefully then woke up barfing. I knew I would forget things but forgetting to burp the baby? It didn't take many throw ups for me to remember to always burp the baby!

Your Child Is Perfect

Every parent thinks and probably says out loud as often as possible – my child is perfect. And they are. Be proud of the breathing, burping, peeing, pooping, sleeping angel that is your child. If you worry that you may not be able to love another child as much as you loved the first – don't. The love is there.

I distinctly remember watching Jett sleeping in my arms. I smelled his sour breath, pulled his long curls and thought to myself, how can I ever love someone as much as I love this little human being? I felt a deep heaviness on my heart because I was scared that having a second child would change the way I felt about Jett. It sounds awful, but I can't deny that I was overwhelmed with such love for Jett that I wondered if there would be enough love for another perfect human being. But there was enough. More than enough. There were times when I felt afraid of having too much love for our kids. Afraid of the energy, strength and power of love that I would have to produce, give and, ultimately, receive. It was scary.

When I was pregnant with Jett, I did a lot of soul-searching and working on my *self*. I felt like I needed to re-confirm who I was. Becoming a mother would be the biggest event in my life. I needed to figure out what I truly believed in and stood for on a core level. I wanted to be ready for all the big questions our kid(s) would ask me. I wanted to make decisions from the foundational place where my truth, knowledge, wisdom and unconditional love lived. I needed to cultivate this place. Of course, life brings on changes that sometimes affect your core beliefs, so this place you make decisions from has to be flexible and prepared for the shifts that may occur. While we all agree that our children are born perfect, I knew that I was not.

I loved Miller before she was fertilized in my womb. When we finally met each other face to face, my love for her gushed out of me like she did, mostly painlessly, easily and beautifully. Loving more than one child was like breathing. It was instinctive and natural. Sometimes overwhelming, but perfect.

The "What If" Questions

The time came during each pregnancy when we had to decide if we would have an amniocentesis test. This test takes a sample of amniotic fluid from your uterus and identifies if your baby has a genetic disorder like Down's Syndrome or Spina Bifida. It's an amazing test in the grand scheme of technological advancement. However, despite the availability of such a test, we decided against taking it each time. We would love whatever perfect child was growing within me. While the decision to say no to the test wasn't a cause for pause, the conversation it created was. "What if" questions certainly arose during both pregnancies.

I can remember when we decided to start trying to get pregnant the first time; I had a moment, a huge cry-hard moment while I was taking a shower. I was naked more than just literally. I thought about the possibility of giving birth to a child with special needs. In fact, my usually loud and busy mind was completely void of anything but this thought. Standing firmly on the folds of my brain was one important question: Will you be okay if you have a child with special needs? The question stood there with her hands on her hips, looking at me, waiting for an answer.

Would I? It was never a question I had to seriously contemplate before. I knew I needed to because anything was possible. I let the hot water pound on my back as I searched within the deepest parts of my heart and soul for a response. Would I be okay if I gave birth to a child with special needs? I felt fear. I felt guilt. I felt anger. I felt love. In that order.

I felt fear because I was afraid that I wouldn't be okay. Maybe I wouldn't be able to care for a special needs child. Then I felt guilty for thinking that I couldn't. I was a walking, talking billboard for unconditional love; how could I think that I'd be too scared to not care for a child that we created? What followed was anger. It fueled the questions: Why me? Why would I get a special needs child? Why couldn't I have a "normal" child?

I needed to know that I would be able to answer these questions and live not with anger, but with love. So I felt the anger. And I cried. I cried because for the first time since we decided to have a baby, I was feeling and thinking like a mother.

I can't even write this section without stopping to move tears out of my blurring eyes. Every parent has to face the "what if" questions. I was overwhelmed with emotions. I felt a heavy hand pushing on my heart. I knew it was Love. She was giving me CPR, gently pumping strength into my heart, sweetly breathing courage into my soul.

As I cried the answers flowed out of me like tears. Yes. Yes, of course I would be able to take care of a child with special needs. I would be able to love any child – in whatever capacity of "normal" that meant.

The possibility of having a child with special needs arose in my mind when I was pregnant the second time. With it the emotions and questions resurfaced. I thought of my good friends Karen and Chris who have an amazing son with Down's Syndrome, Andrew. He is the most loving young man I know. No 19-year old can give a hug like Andrew can. They are a family that is the essence of unconditional love. My emotions about having a special needs child were positive and my answers remained the same when I was pregnant with Miller. I understood completely that we were blessed to have the children we had.

A Crappy Reality

I have an Inflammatory Bowel Disease (IBD) called Ulcerative Colitis (UC). It's a disease that can be dormant until aggravated by things like stress or food. Doctors aren't sure what causes it. I was diagnosed in 1998 after my first year of university. I had just turned twenty. I was living out west in Kelowna, British Columbia and having the time of my life.

Previously in my life, if I ever felt stress I felt it in my guts. I'd have to poo. My mother is the same, and so is her mother. As long as I've been aware of my body's reaction to stress, I've had a nervous stomach, gas and painful poops. When I was living out west, I felt the healthiest and happiest I'd ever been. I never had a nervous stomach. I wasn't feeling any stress. I was excited about life and what I was doing. The doctors told me they didn't know what exactly had caused my flare up.

What was happening inside was this: my immune system thought that the mucus lining my colon was bad. So it started to attack it causing ulcers to form in my colon. They call this a 'flare up' when the intestines get inflamed or full of ulcers. It made me have to poo all the time. And it hurt. A lot. I couldn't keep anything I ate in my system for longer than half an hour. My poo was bloody and when the flare up got severe, my bowel movements were all blood. It was a really shitty situation.

How did the doctors figure all this out? Well, several of them slipped on a rubber glove and shoved a finger up there to feel what was going on. The physical and emotional pain attached to this part of the process still gives me aftershocks. I also had to have several colonoscopies whereby an air blower and a camera were jammed up my butt to take pictures of my colon. Gross. I know. Come the end of the summer after my first year of university, I had come home not with my tail between my legs but with a disease. I had been hospitalized, pumped full of anti-inflammatories, steroids and hope for a stress-free life.

I got through university having several small flare-ups and only one other severe case that landed me in the hospital. Post-university life, I had somehow figured out how to maintain a level of stress that didn't make me sick. I had even made it through my wedding without an ulcer in sight!

I hadn't had a flare up in years. I forgot I even had the disease. So when I arrived home from the hospital with Jett, I wasn't quite sure why my guts were hurting so badly or why I was pooping so much. I attributed it to having just been through twenty-seven hours of labour. In hindsight, I imagine that the stress of my labour was indeed a factor in making the flare up worse, but I'm pretty sure it started in my last months of pregnancy. I had just thought the pain in my guts was from being pregnant. I had been

Life Changes - Again

wrong. It was from both.

Jett and I had spent the first six months of his life in two rooms – the bedroom and the bathroom. They were across the hall from each other (phew). I had been determined to breastfeed, sleep when Jett slept, eat healthy and try to live the life I lived before he was born – cooking, cleaning, exercising. Yeah right. I had gotten a big, fat, bloody piece of reality pie when my specialist told me I was in the middle of a severe flare up. I hadn't wanted to go to the hospital but that's right where I was headed.

I had wanted to continue nursing but the stress it was putting on my body and mind wasn't helping me get better. My energy had been so low, I was barely able to hold Jett. We mostly lay on the bed and played. If I was home alone, I carried Jett into the bathroom with me, sat on the toilet and cried as I had a painful bowel movement. Family members did their best to help us out. If someone could come over and watch Jett so I could sleep, they would. But even sleep wasn't helping enough. The disease would wake me up and I'd have to rush to get to the bathroom. I was averaging six to nine bowel movements a day and I was barely eating.

In July, eight weeks after Jett was born, I was admitted into the hospital with a severe flare up. It was one of the hardest things I'd ever done in my life – leave my family and sleep in a hospital while my two-month old and my husband were at home. It was devastating. I wasn't supposed to be sick. I wasn't supposed to be unable to do all the things I so dearly wanted to. Like hold my child.

Each day in the hospital I'd yearn for Jett. I wanted to hold him and love him. I had to stop nursing as soon as I got to the hospital because of the medicine I had to take and because I physically wasn't there to nurse him. He took to the bottle easily, which I was very thankful for. I cried a lot. I prayed a lot. I hoped I would get better as soon as possible so I could get stronger and go home.

I was pumped full of drugs including Prednisone, a steroid that made me look like I was about to burst. My skin became tight and my cheeks looked like they were full of food. My neck and shoulders looked like someone had plugged a hose into me and filled me up with water. I never looked in the mirror while I was healing. If I had, I wouldn't have left the house. Even though I looked like I'd burst at any moment, the steroids had made the ulcers in my guts slowly disappear.

I also had to have three enemas a day while I was in the hospital. Yup. Three. Morning, noon and night. As the enemas were inserted into my bum hole (one was a bag of medication, the other a bottle), the medication went right to the source of the problem. That's why I had to have so many. Bastards. I was sent home with directions to do two a day until my doctor said to stop. Ugh. One less enema a day but still dreadful. My dear hubby helped me do them. I wasn't able to do them myself both for physical and mental reasons. It's true love when your partner jams medicine up your butt twice a day. True love.

After almost two weeks in the hospital, a nutritionist came in to tell me that I needed to get some fat in my system when I was released. She said I should eat a few Whoppers and Big Macs. I think those were some of the best words I'd heard during that experience!

When I reflect back on the first eight months of Jett's life (that's how long it took me to feel 100% better), I don't know how I did it. I went to a psychic and she told me that I almost died during this flare up, I was so sick. It was funny, I felt like I was dying while I was in the hospital, but I told my body there was no damn way that I was going to die. I was extremely scared, especially during the day when I was alone in my hospital room feeling the disease. Being sick after Jett was born was an experience I wouldn't forget.

When we were ready to start trying for another baby, I was still taking anti-inflammatories. I stayed on certain medications for over a year. I met with my specialist often and we kept a close eye on my condition. We would not let me get sick again. When I did get pregnant I listened to my body. Until I was eight months pregnant I stayed on certain medications. I was as preventative as I could be. I even did some research on UC and pregnancy and learned a lot about what could have potentially caused the flare up while I was pregnant with Jett. I also learned that it's more difficult for women with an IBD to get pregnant.

If you have an IBD or know someone who does, check out www.ccfc.ca to get information about preventative measures to keep your guts healthy and strong during your pregnancy and after. Happy pooping!

Clean Purge Prepare

It was important to me to love the space I lived in. Especially when I was raising children. We lived in a quaint red brick house while we were pregnant with Miller. We lived there until she was a year old and it was the best place we could have been. It was affordable and spacious, my grandparents lived across the street and we could walk to work or daycare. Even though it wasn't our dream house, it was a good home. I liked being there. I felt safe.

When I was six months pregnant with Jett, we moved from a tiny one-bedroom apartment that always smelled like roasted peppers to a bigger apartment because there was no room for the upcoming baby. Needless to say, I couldn't smell or eat peppers without gagging at all during both pregnancies.

We moved to a two-bedroom apartment that was nice, but it was in one of the worst neighbourhoods in the city. It was all that we could afford at the time. We had to choose size over location. When I had been inside the space, I liked it well enough. The two bedrooms were upstairs, and so was the bathroom. The closeness of the bathroom to the bedroom was heaven sent because when we brought Jett home, and I had a brutal ulcerative colitis flare up, I needed the bathroom as close to me as possible.

We promised ourselves that by the time we had our next baby, we'd be living in the house of our dreams. We didn't quite get that far, but the little red brick house we moved to before we were pregnant with Miler was perfect for the time being. It was certainly better than the crack neighborhood apartment as I so aptly named it. It was home sweet home, almost.

It didn't matter what living space I was in, my instinct to "nest" or prepare for the new baby was strong. In fact, it came early and with a ferocious energy when I was pregnant the second time. As soon as I saw the plus sign on the pregnancy stick, I felt the need to clean, purge and re-organize. There were several reasons for this. At work, we were scheduled to do a twenty-one day shoot for a feature film. My role in this endeavour was production manager. This meant that I was responsible for what happened on set everyday. From food to wardrobe to locations, I had to make sure that everyone and everything was in the right place at the right time. This meant that if there was a problem with anything, it was up to me to fix it.

I worked my butt off while Jett was in daycare four days a week. I promised myself that I would do my best to not work when Jett and I had our day together on Fridays. I didn't want to be distracted, but instead dedicate my time and energy to him. We all knew that soon enough there would be another person in the house with whom to share our time, space and energy.

Knowing that the film was happening the last month of my pregnancy meant that I had to have everything in the house ready *before* filming started. I made changes in the house right away. Our bedroom was large enough to use half as a nursery. I dragged the change table, crib parts, baby clothes and necessities out of storage and got right to work. Poor Nick had to build the crib twice. The first time, he put it together in Jett's room. Then we had to take it apart because we couldn't get it through our bedroom door. Ah, the joys of parenthood.

It was important to me that I was able to lie in my bed each night, look across the room where the baby's space was set up and dream about the sweet child who would sleep in the crib. I wanted all the blankets and clothes washed and put away. I wanted the diapers and wipes in baskets beside the change table. I wanted to be ready.

As I was doing laundry for baby number two, I remembered doing laundry for Jett. I had been so overwhelmed after my baby shower. Friends and family gifted us so much stuff and I hadn't been able to wrap my head around using it all. I had wanted to savour the moments of folding and putting the clothes away, decorating the walls in the room and arranging all the stuffed animals perfectly.

I wasn't overwhelmed at all about the baby's space when I was pregnant with Miller. I was prepared. I knew all the stuff we needed. I knew how many washcloths it would take, how many burping blankets. One thing we had that we didn't have with Jett was a glider rocking chair. We got one for Miller. It was amazing. I finished nesting as soon as I could and enjoyed looking at and being in our home and nursery.

Second Baby Go-Aheads

The ten-second rule becomes the however-many-seconds-it-takes-for-me-or-the-child-to-pick-it-up rule when it comes to dropping anything on the floor with baby number two. Food, clothing, toys; it didn't really matter. All the uptight, worried-about-germs paranoia I had oozed when Jett was born was pretty much pushed out in the delivery room when Miller was born.

When it came to worrying about germs and being safe, the second baby was born into adventureland. I'm certainly not saying that we didn't childproof the house. Actually, we hadn't 'unchildproofed' it from when we had done it for Jett. We still closed all the doors behind us, had those get-your-finger-stuck-in-them cupboard locks and a gate that no one ever knew how to open or lock in every doorway possible. I mean, when Miller picked up a piece of hard, dried macaroni and cheese off the floor from yesterday's dinner and put it in her mouth, I didn't freak out. I stuck my hand in her mouth and took it out.

I didn't freak out when Miller pulled out the dining room chair and climbed up so she could lift herself onto the table. Nor did I get nervous when I went into her room and noticed that her bedroom light was on and that her Dora chair was neatly pushed up against the wall beneath the light switch. Oh no. I simply asked her if she turned the light on and when she told me yes, I asked her how. When she climbed up on the chair like a professional circus performer and turned on the light – what did I do? I walked to Nick and told him that Miller could turn her own light on.

Friends that don't have kids often asked me how I was so calm while the kids went bonkers all the time. I told them it wasn't always this way. I wasn't always this calm, and that it wasn't necessarily always calmness that kept me, well, calm, but rather exhaustion. I couldn't add a layer of paranoia to my already loaded shoulders, I told them. I watched the kids and did my best to stop them from engaging in dangerous acts, but I wasn't as afraid of them falling or getting hurt.

The first six to eight months as a first-time parent, I had been extremely paranoid. I made everyone wash their hands before they held Jett. I wouldn't let anyone put anything in their mouth if it could potentially go into Jett's mouth (like a spoon or a soother). I washed toys like they were covered in the plague. I never purposefully let Jett fall. I say purposefully because there was one time when he was two months old that he fell…off the counter… onto the kitchen floor…while he was in a baby chair. If I could have avoided it, I would have. But I couldn't. I watched him slow motion fall from the counter, landing head first on the kitchen floor making a sound that no parent should ever have to hear.

Why had he been in his chair on the counter? I didn't think he could move it. He shifted. It moved. He fell. Before he let out the first guttural wail there was a moment of silence as there often is when kids fall. Like the fall itself, this moment was also in slow motion. As he bawled, I held him to my heart and apologized.

Kids are resilient and pretty much made of rubber. They are meant to fall and hurt themselves and learn to not do whatever it was that caused them pain. As a parent, I learned very quickly where *not* to put an infant no matter how sturdy I think he or his seating device may be.

By the time Jett learned how to walk, which was about ten months, I had to give up my über paranoia that he would get hurt or catch some ghastly germ disease. Once he had mastered his mobility, I had lost most, if not all, of my control over him getting hurt. The amazing thing was that the more freedom I gave him to learn to fall and get up, and fall and get up the more confident he became. He never hurt himself badly, and if something caused him to cry, it usually wasn't because he hurt himself, but because it frightened him. We would talk about what happened so he understood that what he did made him hurt himself, and then he would try not to do it again.

With Miller, she was like a little dog that thought she was a big dog. She saw Jett climb up on the couch and throw his head into the pillows and she wanted to do it too. She was a daredevil by instinct and default. She put everything into her mouth. Jett never did. She loved to eat paper. Sometimes, I just let her eat it. She'd poop it out.

Most of the time, whatever she put in her mouth, she took out and handed to me anyway. I'd get a palm full of thick globs of wet cardboard chewed off all the cards from Jett's board games or chunks of dried food. She knew she wasn't supposed to eat those things. We would tell her no, she would make her choice and we'd deal with the consequences.

Miller ate her first french fry before she was a year old. As soon as she switched to solid food, french fries were in the mix. At first, we'd give her one or two. She was eating chopped up pieces of what we were eating quite early in her big people food-eating career. She didn't like baby food so we chopped and smooshed what we were eating and she was happy with this.

Jett hadn't had his first french fry until he was almost three years old, at least that we knew about. Even at age three, we had been very apprehensive about giving him fast food. We hadn't wanted him to know what McDonald's was, and we certainly didn't want him to ask for it all the time. Well, after Miller was born, he quickly learned what McDonald's was and he loved it. In fact, he told us his favorite food was a hamburger.

We didn't want our kids to be fast food kids, but that meant we couldn't be fast food parents. Before we even thought about it, we went through a drive-thru and handed Miller some fries. She was halfway through a Chicken McNugget Kid's Meal before I even realized what we'd done – tainted our child with the delicious food stylings of Mr. Ronald McDonald.

Some of the beliefs we stood our ground on with the first child got gooey when the second child came along. We opted for easier over healthier. But we were conscious of it so we did our best to not do it frequently.

The ability to make a positive choice is one of the best things we can teach our children. I've learned that we have to promise that if we teach and give our children the ability to choose well, and we positively respond to the consequences of their choices, they'll make good choices. This knowledge solidified when Miller was born. When she put that first chunk of mystery-dried food into her sweet, drooling mouth, I had to decide if I was going to freak out in a paranoid, irrational way or not. I chose not. I choose not. I kiss a lot of bumps and bruises. I throw out a lot of mystery food. And it's okay. Our kids are learning how to make good choices thus far.

Date Night

Nick and I found sanctuary in the movie theatre. We both loved films so date night often consisted of a movie, a hump and a talk (sometimes a hump, a movie and a talk). Getting out of the house together was an extremely important thing we promised each other. My friends laughed at me when I'd tell them I was having a "date night" with Nick, but it was the truth. We had to treat it that way so we could keep some sort of fire in our personal relationship. We'd look at the calendar and include a date night with all the other important things – doctor's appointments, work-related things, family events, etc.

We'd get a sitter, chose a movie, and leave early so we could have a quick romp before the film started. We'd buy popcorn, nachos and share a hotdog and a jug of pop, then settle in for a quick escape. After the movie, we'd talk about it on the way home, engaging in the most grown-up conversation we'd had since the last date.

Fitting it all in was a time management nightmare but it wasn't impossible. If Nick and I ever needed to talk about things like a parenting or personal issue, we treated this with the same importance. Got a sitter, had the talk, perhaps made love and went back home. Date nights were something we looked forward to…almost as much as sleep!

Boobs

beautiful breasts

Cleavage itches, stretching skin sensation, sticking out, standing up, yelling hello. Our child will suck on my nipple, milk will come out. Baby's private cow. The water in the shower hits my nipples. I have to turn away. It hurts. We marvel at how big my boobs get and giggle when we see them get bigger. They jiggle when I laugh and this makes us laugh harder. My breasts are not my breasts. Swollen sore, filling puffy pumping veins. Falling down over my heart towards you.

In the morning, fresh with rest, when we don't miss each other yet, he cups my swelling breast, kisses the green-blue-purple veins spidering to my puffy nipples.

Mom Boobs

I had great tits before I had kids. I liked them a lot. They measured in at a perky and round 34B. I could get away with going braless in public, and my knockers still looked sexy. At the time, of course, I took them and their beautiful magnitude for granted. During the course of both pregnancies, my breasts went from B cups to DD to C and finally back to B. It took almost four years to get them back to their original size.

In their naked state, they hang low with strong potential for wobbling to and fro. There is no perkiness anywhere. They hang flat against my chest with white stretch marks aiming down toward my nipples that reach mid ribs. When I lie on my back, they fall to the sides and play hide-and-seek with my armpits. When erect, my nipples still look and feel good.

Sometimes Nick says, "You've got beautiful boobs, baby." It's very nice of him to say. He likes them well enough. And that matters especially when I lift them up off my ribs and ask "why?" I'm thankful they still work! Miller loves my boobs too. When she has a bottle or is sleepy, she slips her hand down my shirt and holds my nipple, not caring at all how low they hang.

I knew this change would happen. I'd seen mom boobs before. I'd seen the fall. But I secretly told myself, *not my boobs*. Yeah right, I totally have mom boobs. After ballooning out to size double-baby-head, as we used to joke when feeding Miller, it's no wonder they pulled and stretched and fell to the ground.

To Boob Or To Bottle?

Before we became pregnant with Jett, I had an opinion about breastfeeding. I wanted to breastfeed but I wasn't opposed to using formula if it was necessary. I treated this decision-making process like I treated the epidural – I'd do what I could with all my heart and might until I needed help. The same went for baby #2.

As planned, I began nursing Jett when he was born. I did it until I couldn't anymore because my ulcerative colitis was in a terrible flare up. I had to decide if I was going to let myself get sicker and stay nursing or start taking medicine and use formula. I had to choose getting better because if I wasn't healthy enough to take care of my own body, how was I supposed to take care of a baby? I had to be realistic with my situation even though the new mother in me had wanted to keep nursing.

I breastfed Jett for about eight weeks, and during that time, he latched without a problem. When we took him in for a check-up when he was a few days old, the nurse told us that he'd lost weight because he wasn't getting enough milk. We had to supplement with formula a couple of times because he had lost too much weight. We had to feed him with a small syringe. The formula we had was so thick and heavy that after only a few drops, Jett had eaten his fill. He looked like he was blissfully drunk. We had only supplemented a few times before I had enough milk and he gained weight. When it came time to officially switch to formula, Jett didn't have any nipple confusion or attachment issues with the bottle. He had always been hungry and he would eat whatever we gave him.

We tried pre-mixed and powder, but settled on using the just-add-water formula. We tried the powder because it was cheaper, but Jett didn't seem to like it as much. At one point, there were some people in the city who were opening the powder formula and putting laundry detergent into it. Parents were buying it and using it and their kids were getting sick. I just couldn't fathom buying the powder formula after that. It didn't matter how much money we could have saved, even though money was an issue at that time.

When Miller was born, and I knew I wasn't having issues with my ulcerative colitis, I easily slipped into nursing as my feeding choice. I only had a little bit of experience doing it from the first time, but it was enough to give me the confidence that it would work. Miller was nursing well in no time. So much of nursing had to do with my energy. There had to be an air of peace and ease when I did it because Miller felt everything I did. If I was stressed while I was trying to nurse, it was a challenge for her to latch. She could feel my energy.

It was the same when Nick was feeding Miller too. When I couldn't feed and Nick did it, sometimes it was a challenge for him. He didn't think it had anything to do with his energy, but I think it did, especially if I was home at the same time, but was unable to do it myself. If Miller knew I was home, she wanted me to feed her. Nick said it was because she knew I was there, and she wanted the boob not the bottle. If she had her choice it was boob over bottle every time.

Nursing created an undeniable connection between my kids and me. We had to be prepared for this both times. The reality was that Nick and I had to work a bit harder to get Miller to eat, whether I was around to do the feeding or not. I needed his help.

I knew women who came from a long line of formula-feeding mothers. I knew women who were breastfed but decided not to nurse their own children. I was breastfed and so was my mom. I always knew I wanted to breastfeed so when the time came, I did. Choosing to boob or to bottle was a personal choice first and a circumstantial one when the baby came out. No matter what, I had to take it one boob or bottle at a time.

Taste Test

I had to. I just had to taste my breast milk. I waited for the perfect opportunity. It came on a Saturday night when I was going out with my best friend and dancing partner, Linda. It was a full on girls' night. The kind we used to have when we were in university when our toughest choice was whether we should study or dance. It had been ages since we'd gotten together for a night out. We were so excited to eat, drink and dance that we started at her apartment doing all three.

As she danced into her bar clothes, and I, well, just danced, I could feel my boobs filling up with milk. I was still nursing at this point. I knew I would be drinking so I'd have to pump or squeeze out the milk before I fed Miller. Before we left for the restaurant, I needed a little release or my boobs would be squirting out milk all night. I had an idea.

I asked Linda if she had a fancy glass. She handed me a martini glass. In her bathroom, I pulled out a boob and squeezed some milk into it. I did the same with the other boob. When I was finished, I had filled about half the martini glass. We both looked at it and burst out laughing. I asked her if she wanted a shot. She declined. I understood.

Before I took a sip, I asked myself – *what are you doing?* My answer came quickly – *tasting it*. I'd wanted to taste it since I started nursing. I produced the milk, so it couldn't be unhealthy to drink. It couldn't taste that bad; Miller couldn't keep her mouth away from it. I didn't want to think too hard about the psychological implications of what I was about to do.

In my head I kept it light and before I could chicken out I put the glass to my lips and took a sip. It was surprisingly warm, much warmer than I expected. I laughed out loud. Linda asked me what it tasted like. I told her it was really sweet. I couldn't remember what I'd eaten that day, but by the taste of the milk, it was like all I had eaten was sugar. It was thinner in consistency than I imagined. I thought it would be thicker like a milk shake. It felt slick in my mouth. I quickly figured out what it reminded me of: it felt like semen. It stayed warm in my throat like a shot. I couldn't drink it all. I looked at what was left in the glass. I swished it around, said goodbye and poured it down the sink.

I don't know what possessed me to do it aside from pure curiosity. I offered it to Nick once but he declined. One day I lifted my nipple up to see if it would reach my mouth. It did, but I couldn't bring myself to take a sip. When I got home from my girls' night, I told Nick that I had tasted my breast milk. He asked me if it was good. I told him it was different than I expected. I'm glad I did it. I didn't think it was gross. It quenched my curiosity. I'll admit it may have been a bit dramatic to put it into a martini glass, but it was actually perfect too. A Milky Martini.

Leaky Loo

My boobs leaked milk all the time. At night. During the day. In between feedings. If Miller didn't eat as much or if I wasn't with her and missed a feeding, they leaked even more. I'd feel a surge of wet heat at my nipple. I'd look down and see a round, whitish circle of wetness seeping through my shirt. Breast pads, you ask? Where were the breast pads? I tried using them. I really did. But they made my boobs look ridiculous. It didn't matter what bra I wore or which brand of pads I used, I looked like I had a round diaper over each nipple. So I used tissue instead. It wasn't as thick but it was enough to catch the initial leakage and I would attend to the matter by feeding Miller, expressing milk or pumping.

Since I breastfed way longer with Miller and was producing milk at what seemed like a ridiculously rapid rate, leaking happened more with the second baby than it did with the first. In fact, I hadn't leaked at all when I was nursing Jett. I don't think I had produced enough milk to leak so much. I hadn't leaked before either child was born. I'd heard that some women's breasts filled with milk before they went into labour. This hadn't happened to me.

I remember being out on a date with Nick. His

mom got us tickets to go see Hall & Oates. We went out for a fancy dinner at an Italian restaurant. I had one glass of wine and was tipsy and happy. We arrived at the venue on time and sat to enjoy the music. I felt a subtle surge of warmth in my bra but I had put tissue over my nipples so I assumed I was covered. As the show progressed, however, my boobs started to get bigger. I could literally feel the milk pumping out of my glands. The high-pitched cooing of Darryl Hall didn't help. I think my body thought it was a baby crying, not a grown man singing in wicked falsetto.

    I was thankful when the lights came up. I had to pee and my boobs were sobbing in pain. I happened to look down. There were two huge white circles on my chest. I laughed out loud. Nick looked at me. I pointed at my boobs. "Thirsty?" I asked him. I had leaked through the tissue onto my fancy black shirt. Nice. Thank goodness I brought a scarf. I placed it strategically so to hide my leaky loo boobs. It wasn't the first time I'd leak in public. And it wouldn't be the last.

Cold Turkey Boobs

I breastfed much longer than I ever thought I would. I thought I would maybe nurse for eight months – max. But eight months rolled around like the extra bum above my hamstrings and I just couldn't do it. I loved nursing. I loved holding Miller up close to me and watching her nestling into my giant boobs. I loved the way she would fondle and flick the nipple of the boob she wasn't using like she owned it and could do what she wanted to it. She pulled, smacked, fondled, held, hugged and squeezed my boobs. I loved looking down at her as she was feeding. The way she would get thrilled at the sight of my boob as I unfolded it out of my bra and shirt. Nursing came naturally to us. It was free, convenient and mostly painless. Not to mention, it was a tremendous bonding experience… wait, why would I want to stop doing this?

The truth was that something in me knew it was time to stop. Miller was fifteen months old. Her first birthday had come and gone. I told myself on several occasions that I was going to stop. I bought 9 oz. bottles and found our bottle warmer. I told Nick I was going to stop, but then I never did. I was even down to only nursing at bedtime and once during the night. I thought I wasn't producing that much milk anymore. My boobs were big, but they were squishy during off time so I didn't think it would be difficult to stop. Miller had four teeth – two up and two down. She bit me on three separate occasions. When she did, I screamed and yanked her off and it scared us both.

The winter holidays arrived and I was ready to stop nursing – for real. This time when I told Nick I was stopping, he knew I meant it. It meant that I would need extra support at bedtime. He needed to be on the proverbial bandwagon with me. I couldn't do it alone.

Even though I was a wreck inside, and I felt bad for taking away something Miller obviously loved so much, I knew it was time. I felt like I was being a tough mother. I thought Miller would get angry with me and not take a bottle. It was an emotional time for me, certainly one of the biggest challenges of being a mother.

I think it was the long stretch of holidays that gave me the strength to stop almost stopping and really do it. So one day, I just stopped. Specifically, December 21st. Feeding time came. We laid down together on the bed. I offered her a bottle and she took it. No problem. She immediately went to grab my boobs. I let her. She looked at them, then up at me. I said as sweetly as I could without crying, "All done!" Miller repeated after me, "All done?" I told her again, "All done!" She looked at my boobs questioningly then she went back to the bottle. No crying. No squirming. No problem.

I was so relieved. After that night, the switch continued to go smoothly. She looked at my boobs lustfully, but didn't actually try to drink from them anymore. She did, however, continue to fondle, smack, grab and handle them, my nipples especially. In fact, even if I picked her up or held her, she'd sneak her little hand down my shirt and grab a boob.

I did research about what would happen when I stopped and the best way to stop so it wasn't painful. I bought a giant cabbage. I'd been told to put cold cabbage leaves over my boobs because they helped soothe the pain and they sucked up the milk. I did this once or twice at night. It didn't get stinky, which I was also told might happen.

During the last weeks of nursing, my boobs didn't get hard or sore. I thought they were only filling at night when I needed the milk. But I was wrong. Just because they were squishy and not rock hard didn't mean there wasn't milk in them. There was.

When the second night of not feeding rolled around, my boobs were so huge, full and hard I couldn't move. I couldn't sleep. To look at them was painful. Several times a night, I leaned over the bathroom sink and expressed milk from each boob to take the pressure off. I started at the top of my boob and gently pressed my fingers down toward my nipple. The pain was the worst at the tops and the sides, so that's where my hand went first. I did this until the pressure subsided. Sometimes it took about fifteen minutes to get both boobs expressed enough that it didn't hurt when I breathed. I cried a lot.

Some websites said to pump, but to be careful to only pump enough to stop the pressure. I didn't do this. I didn't want to risk pumping too much and making more milk, and I couldn't find my pump anyway. All the websites said to wean the baby off the boob, to gradually decrease my amount of milk production. I thought I did that by only feeding Miller in the evening and at night, but if I went by the pain I was having, and by the ridiculous amount of milk my boobs were still producing, I guess I didn't wean enough. This meant I stopped nursing pretty much cold turkey. It was painful.

It took about three weeks for my boobs to be completely empty. Then they shrunk and I was happy. It was nice to not have two basketball-sized boobs on my chest every day. They also fell. Down. Way down. To mid-belly. Ugh. Gone was the perk that I so happily enjoyed.

I had so many stretch marks it looked like someone painted light purple lines all over each boob. And they were very squishy to touch. They felt kind of like chunks of wet Cheez Whiz. But look, it wasn't anything a good bra couldn't handle.

Vagina 101

my girl

Little, quiet, sometimes shy. Luscious, juicy, sour sweet. My girl likes to be touched. She's been scrubbed rubbed ripped and repaired. Poked stroked fingered and fondled. She responds to me, my man and others. Sometimes just by thinking, looking, dreaming. She hopes and requests, welcomes and receives.

My friend, my self, my soul, a perfectly unique satisfyingly beautiful hole. With a twist of lust, a reddish, warm embrace.

Changes To My Girl

My vagina was sore during my whole second pregnancy. She was under a lot of pressure, quite literally. I wondered how she would change this time around. I didn't worry that she would be loose, which seemed like a bit of a concern among some of the women I spoke to. I knew from the first pregnancy that my girl was very powerful. She had undergone a twenty-seven hour delivery, layers of stitches and she healed up pretty well. She never went back to how she was before I delivered, but she made it through the pain and still worked.

In the hospital, minutes after Jett was born, I had propped myself up in the bed and noticed the doctor's head poking up between my legs. I peered over and watched him pulling a thick thread up with tweezers. I asked him what he was doing. He told me he was stitching me up. I asked him if it was bad, and he told me that I ripped from my vagina to my bum. "I stopped it just before your hole," he said. I leaned back on the bed, thankful that I couldn't feel what he was doing. He stitched for over twenty minutes.

After eight weeks of healing had passed, and the stitches and the pain dissipated, my girl had been in a state that was ready for lovin' again. But she felt different. Not to the touch on the outside, but on the inside when having sex. She had been tighter, not looser. My perineum (the place between where the vagina ends and the bum hole starts) felt tighter. It had been way more sensitive and, during sex, more pleasurable.

Pre-pregnancy, my girl had been like a rose in full bloom. Post-pregnancy, she had been like a rose that couldn't quite spread her petals. When having sex, it felt like there was only a certain way Nick's penis could go in or else it felt like it was hitting something. When I had talked to my OB/GYN about it, she suggested that it was scar tissue. This had made sense to me. It felt like there was a soft wall that didn't want to allow anything through. If there had been scar tissue built up inside, it made sense that it would feel like the sides of my vagina were blocking the entrance.

Compared to Jett's labour, Miller's was heavenly. I only needed a few stitches, and there wasn't any tearing to my perineum. My vagina healed much quicker. When Nick and I had sex, it was painful but not as painful as it was after Jett was born. That blocked feeling I had felt while having sex was there again but not as intense. It felt like my vagina wasn't fully awake yet. You know in the morning, if you give yourself time to have those few giant, invigorating stretches, how much more awake you feel? It felt like my vagina needed to have an invigorating morning stretch. As time passed, and as only time can allow, my girl healed up nicely. She made the stretch. My vagina is resilient. I would never underestimate her.

A Girl And A Mirror

I had looked at my vagina once after Jett was born. What was crazy was that I didn't remember until looking back in my journal and found an entry about me taking a peek. It was about eight weeks after I'd given birth. All I wrote was that she didn't *look* different.

People that know me will tell you I'll talk about anything. *Anything.* My girlfriends will tell you that they're totally surprised to know that I've never had alone time with my girl and a mirror. The truth is I'm shy. I'm shy about my girl. I don't really want to look at her. I know she's there. I know she works. I know I can touch her and it feels good. I know Nick can touch her and it feels good. I know she's small and kind of hidden.

But, every woman has a special relationship with her vagina whether she looks at her with a mirror or not. When you have a baby so much of your journey is in relation to your vagina. The whole process is miraculous. I can only believe that my girl could stretch that much because I have two children as proof. I am amazed that she still works after all that has passed through her.

Scent Of A Woman

During both pregnancies, one of the things that I experienced was an intensified sense of smell. This didn't bode well as it made me become increasingly paranoid about how my vagina smelled. There were some days when all I could smell was the sour sweet scent of my consistently discharging vagina. I kept asking my mom and sister, "Can you smell it? Can you smell my vagina?" They always said no. I hoped they were telling the truth.

While no one wants to talk about it and, most importantly, smell it, the truth is that each vagina has a scent. This scent changes when you're pregnant. The smell of my vagina during pregnancy changed all the time. The amount of stuff coming out of my vagina changed each week, even each day, toward the end.

The attention given to my girl became greater and greater as my due dates approached. When the mucus plug came out, it came out of the vagina. When the water broke, it broke out of the vagina. There was so much action going on around my girl that I just had to pay more attention to her.

Discharge. It's such an awful term. I find so many words related to the vagina don't match the beauty that it is. Discharge sounds so medical and distant, like something that comes out of a car engine or a machine. Clitoris. It sounds too hard and tough when in reality it's soft and gentle. Vulva, now that's more like it. Vulva is the word for all the external female genitals. We don't use this word often though, do we? I'm just saying…

Treats. That's what I called my discharge. I had crazy treats in my undies each day when I was pregnant. My doctor said that as long as it wasn't green or bloody, treats were natural, normal and plentiful. Now treats, like semen, don't easily come out of material, so I had to get rid of a bunch of underwear. I waited until about eight weeks after Miller came home to buy new ones though. Post-pregnancy treats are as plentiful as during. Enjoy shopping for new underwear when the time comes.

There was something that helped save my undergarments from the onslaught of discharge: pads or tissues. I was a tissue girl. I had tried wearing mini-pads over the years. I tried all different brands and thicknesses during my first pregnancy. I remember standing in the feminine needs aisle at the grocery store, sweating a bit and staring blankly at the wall of boxes. Wings. Weaves. Light days. Heavy days. I was in a daze. It had been crazy trying to figure out which box to buy. I tried everything.

I just couldn't find a pad that fit me well. It always scrunched up or unstuck, and the seam at the back end always gave me a rash in my bum crack. So I opted against mini-pads. I used tissues. I took two tissues, folded them in half and gently laid them in my undies. Regular, on sale, no fancy added cream tissues.

They were soft, reliable, and the perfect thickness. Every time I went to the bathroom, I changed the tissues. If there were no tissues available, a double layer of a few squares of toilet paper was always a great cover. If I wasn't washing everyday but was changing my undies, I for sure needed some tissue to help absorb the scent and the treats my lovely girl was giving me.

MacGyver Mom

Note to pregnant self: wash my girl before all doctor's appointments. This way I'm safe. I'm clean. I'm ready. Of course, sometimes there just wasn't time to do a quick refresher down there. Anyone could argue that cleaning my girl was something to make time to do. I could assure you, however, that these 'anyones' have never been nine months pregnant and caring for a toddler. In any case, if I could, I tried to do a quick wash up before I went to the OB/GYN especially at the end of the pregnancy because I'd probably have to have an internal exam at every visit.

During my first pregnancy I had been on it. I was totally aware of all the procedures that would happen at the doctor's office. I asked questions. I took notes. Nick and I went together. I had been as keen as a brownnoser the first day of class. With Miller, I knew I needed internal exams; however, I forgot at what point they happened.

One such visit to my OB/GYN, I was taken to an exam room, and told to undress from the waist down. I remember chuckling to myself as I realized that this would be a visit with an internal exam. I hadn't washed my girl since the day before. In the morning. I was going on what

I called 'day-old vagina.' I knew it wasn't the most pleasant place to be poking around in its present state.

I surveyed the room. A sink. Some antibacterial hand soap. Paper towels. Perfect. I took off my shoes, pants and undies as quickly as I could. I went to the sink, grabbed some paper towels, wet them with warm water, squirted them with soap, and quickly washed my girl. Of course, in mid scrub, I heard a gentle tap on the door. I hooted, "Just a minute!" I did a quick rinse, then a quick dry. I smooshed my wet paper towel deep into the garbage so the doctor wouldn't see any evidence of my secret cleaning. I scooted up onto the examination table, white paper crunching beneath my naked bum. It wasn't fully dry so the paper was sticking to my butt cheek as I tried to lie down.

I said, "I'm ready," to no one. Since I hadn't answered right away, the doctor had moved on to her next patient. I'd lost my place in line, but it was okay. I'd managed to clean my girl. I waited, laughing at myself, but not without a little MacGyver-ish pride.

The Practice Vagina

At my doctor's office, a few days before I was due for Miller, I went in for my weekly check-up. I got naked from the waist down, climbed up on the uncomfortable examination table, made a crinkling symphony trying to get into a comfortable position and waited. I remembered I was having an internal exam at this visit, so my girl was squeaky clean. Since I knew I was going to have an internal exam, I wanted to lie down and relax as much as I could so my girl wouldn't tighten up for the ol' plunge.

A male intern came in first. Young. Eager. Friendly. He asked me a bunch of questions. We had a pretty lengthy conversation about discharge. Lovely. He measured my belly. We listened to the baby's galloping heartbeat. He told me he would be back in with the doctor. I waited another couple of minutes. They came in and I could tell by the look on the intern's face that something was up. My instincts started whispering.

Now, I really liked my doctor. She was friendly, informative, relaxed and funny. I trusted her. If she asked me to allow the intern to do an internal, I trusted that she believed this person was capable. My instincts were right. It didn't take long before she asked whether I minded if the intern did a checkup after she did hers. I said okay. She pulled on a rubber glove, lubed it up, walked to my legs and spread them open. She apologized as she plunged her fingers deep inside me. She told me I was one centimeter dilated. I couldn't tell at all. The only difference was it didn't feel as tight as the last time she checked me. She took her hand out. The intern was prepped; a rubber glove was lubed up on his hand too. He moved to the table, leaned forward and gently put his fingers inside me. He looked up at the ceiling and tried to avoid eye contact. He looked scared and extremely uncomfortable. I felt like giggling, but I stopped myself. Poor guy.

I could tell that he wasn't inside me nearly as deep as the doctor had been. So I told him, "You gotta push in deeper." The doctor laughed at me. I was trying to make it easier for the intern. Gesturing between the two of us, my doctor described and showed with her fingers what the intern should feel. I told him it was okay, that I thought he was touching and feeling what she was describing. He just kept looking at the ceiling and saying, "I'm not sure if I'm feeling what you're describing." The look of confusion never left his face. He stopped moving his fingers, pulled out his hand, took off the glove and we all felt a bit of relief. The doctor thanked me and so did the intern. Then he shook my hand with the one he'd just used for my internal exam. Fantastic. The practice vagina. That's my girl.

When I had been in labour with Jett, my girl had been the practice vagina for catheter insertion. I was frozen from the waist down from the epidural so I couldn't feel a thing down there. I remember I was lying on my back with my legs spread wide open, a nurse on each side of me. One was teaching, the other was learning. The learning nurse was shy and she looked petrified as the teaching nurse showed her what to do. I smiled in all my epidural glory and told the training nurse to go nuts. Make a mistake. Do it more than once. It didn't bother me 'cause I couldn't feel a thing. They both laughed at me. The training nurse got the catheter in on the first try.

Kegels Shmegels

Would my vagina remember what it felt like being pregnant and how to give birth like the rest of my body? If it would, would it be angry with me for not exercising it like I exercised the rest of my body? If you're like me, you did your best to exercise while you were pregnant the first time. When pregnant with my second, I barely even thought about it. My vagina was in the same boat. I had done Kegels a few times while I was pregnant with Jett and barely thought about doing them while pregnant with Miller.

All the pregnancy books screamed at me to do Kegels and massage my perineum. I understood why. It strengthened the muscles I would use during labour. Got it, but just couldn't *do* it. My vagina was so sore during my second pregnancy that squeezing it consciously for exercise was a torturous idea. As much as I loved the *idea* of Kegels and the secrecy of this exercise, (I'm doing it right now. Nobody knows…) I didn't love how much it hurt to do it.

The other Kegels problem was that not only did they hurt they made me horny, and I ended up masturbating or having sex. I couldn't very well masturbate or have sex all day, now could I? I'm not sure how one measures the strength of her vagina muscles, but when shove had come to push during labour with Jett, it hadn't mattered how strong my girl was. He hadn't wanted to come out and we had to pull him out with forceps. I pushed until I puked and I don't think any amount of Kegels would have helped get him out.

Between My Legs

By the fifth month of pregnancy number two, sleep was difficult. It wasn't because I was exhausted or because Jett was hogging the middle of the bed and either kicking or punching me in his sleep – that was bearable. I couldn't get comfortable. I forgot what side I was supposed to sleep on. I knew not to lie on my back. I remembered that much. Training my body to fall asleep in one position was a challenge. I needed a pillow.

Nick and I each had two pillows for sleeping. I only used one of mine because it supported my head the way I liked. The other one was too soft and often ended up not being used, on the floor or up against the headboard. I decided to make this pillow my crotch pillow. I put an extra pillowcase on it and shoved it between my legs. It was a little piece of crotch heaven.

I told Nick not to use it. It got smelly quickly. The mixture of leg and crotch sweat meant this pillow was not for a head to rest on. The stink was inevitable. So I washed it and put it in the dryer. It weathered that storm. I'd had a crotch pillow while I was pregnant with Jett as well. No matter what kind of pillow you use, I recommend using one. If it finds itself between your legs, so be it.

Positioning during sleep became easier. The crotch pillow enabled me to sleep on my side without hurting my lower back. I left one leg straightened out and the other loosely bent up. The pillow caught my leg and crotch sweat. It was my sleeping saviour.

Self Serve Or On The Side

I was never a huge masturbator. If I had to choose between masturbation and having sex with Nick, I'd choose sex with Nick each time. But when I was pregnant again, things changed in the sex department. I wasn't a particularly horny person to begin with and I wasn't sure how being pregnant would affect my libido. Sexually, Nick and I had always been compatible; our libidos were similar. I didn't become a sex-craved monster while I was pregnant, but I wanted to be able to still do it. Nick wasn't one of those guys who was worried about poking the baby in the head when we had sex, so he was up for it if I was. Thus, I became the dictator of our sex schedule during both pregnancies.

By the time I was seven months with Miller, I couldn't have sex anymore without being in a lot of pain. It felt like someone was stepping on the inside of my vagina. There was a lot of pressure on my girl. If my vagina lips looked like a mouth, they'd be Angelina Jolie's with a lip infusion. They felt huge and sore all the time. I tried. I really tried to do it, but my wincing-in-pain face just wasn't a turn on for Nick, poor guy. I was a bit hornier than usual but not for penetration sex. I opted for masturbation.

Mostly shower masturbation.

In the shower I felt warm and clean. I was alone. I got through my usual shower routine then I had a few special moments with my girl. It didn't take long to reach orgasm and the orgasms always felt fantastic. They relieved pressure on my girl and she felt a little better the few hours after I masturbated.

Sometimes I'd masturbate with my trusty crotch pillow. It was already down there. I did it in bed before I took a nap. Having a quick orgasm always helped me fall asleep and it made my cold feet get warm. I had masturbated while I was pregnant with Jett but not as much as I did when I was pregnant with Miller. I had been able to have sex without pain right up until the end of the pregnancy with Jett. This was one major difference between pregnancy number one and number two.

Nick was extremely supportive of my sex needs or lack thereof. That's not to say we didn't do other things. I remember an influx in the amount of oral sex I provided. I wanted him to feel pleasure somehow, and if it wasn't via vaginal sex then oral sex was the next best thing. He would have returned the favor, but I really didn't want him near my girl with all that was going on with her. The pressure, the discharge; I just didn't think it was a nice place to be.

It wasn't that bad. We were both so tired all the time with work and raising Jett that when we plopped into bed each night, sex wasn't the first thing on our minds – sleep was. They say that having sex can help induce labour. I can't confirm this, but I can tell you that masturbation sure induced feeling good. I've got first-hand experience. No pun intended. Okay, maybe a little.

When we did have sex, the most comfortable position was when I was on my back with my hips to the side. I didn't go on top because I didn't want to weigh Nick down and he didn't go on top because my belly was in the way. Doggy-style was just uncomfortable. I found that if I lie on my back and shifted my hips to the side, and Nick was on his side entering me that way, it was most pleasurable for both of us.

I never had trouble having orgasms, self-given or with Nick. The intensity of my orgasms increased while I was pregnant. They lasted longer and often felt so good I saw stars. After both kids were born, how much sex did we have? On average, about twice a week and that was a good week!

Humping and Jumping

I had been quite open when I told my friends and family that we were trying to get pregnant the first time. I wanted their support in the matter. Nick hadn't liked it as much because if someone asked, and we weren't pregnant then we'd have to tell the person that too. And everyone asked. I still blabbed anyway.

Basically, it meant we told our friends and family we were having lots of sex. Specifically, the kind of sex that would have Nick cumming like mad to get me knocked up. There wouldn't be another situation in my life when I looked at my 83 year-old grandfather and told him, "I'm going to have lots of sex with my husband from now until we get pregnant." That was probably why we said we were 'trying' and not that we were 'humping' or insert your sex word of choice.

When we were trying to get pregnant the first time, I never thought that telling people we were trying meant telling people we were having a lot of sex. I was so caught up in the fact that we were actually going to make and have a baby, I didn't really think about what it meant. The second time, I realized it and said, "Hey, we're humping like rabbits 'cause we wanna make a baby!"

Sex became less than fun when all I thought about while I was doing it was whether or not we'd conceive. When we were trying to get pregnant with Jett, I tried to remember each time, position and feeling I had during sex so I could distinctly remember his conception. What I should have been doing was enjoying how good it felt to hump. I never knew when I was ovulating because my period was inconsistent off the pill. So we had sex all the time.

I coloured a red heart on the calendar each time we made love and a black X when I had my period. The calendar hung in our bedroom, the place we most frequently got it on. It was like a megaphone screaming at us. After the fourth month of not getting pregnant, the process was stifling. Our expectations had deflated at warp speed. We reached a point where we weren't 'making love,' we were sex-bots fueled by grief. The fun had gone.

We had gotten to the point when we just gave up 'trying.' We had sex whenever we felt like it. We said out loud that we didn't care anymore if and when we got pregnant. And mostly, I believed this in my heart. I kept keeping track of things on the calendar, but I hid it so it wasn't in our faces. Sex became making love again, and believe it or not, I actually don't know exactly when Jett was conceived. I'm pretty sure it had been at a party. Sloppy, exciting, boozy baby-making. Lovely. In total, it took us five months to get pregnant for Jett. As soon as we let our expectations go, we got knocked up.

We knew we wanted another baby. I envisioned

having kids close together. My sister and I were only ten months apart. I was used to having a sibling close in age and I wanted the same thing for our kids. Okay, maybe not ten months apart, but close. However, I was told I needed to wait at least two years before we could even start trying because of my ulcerative colitis. Two years was a long time to wait in my plan book.

I'd always been a person who gave herself personal deadlines: sex by eighteen, graduate by early twenties, marry by mid-twenties, babies by thirty. About eighteen months after Jett was born, I felt great and wanted to start trying for baby number two. I met with my doctors and got the go ahead. I promised myself this time would be different. I wouldn't get all stressed out. Well, this was much easier said than done.

While I didn't mark up the calendar, and we weren't having sex all over the place all the time, I did find a new obsession. Pregnancy tests. I swear I peed on a stick every five minutes. After seeing so many negatives, I didn't want to do a test at all. Once again, I had to give it up. Relax. Enjoy the process. Alas, the only way to find out if I was pregnant was to take a test so I couldn't completely escape my obsession.

One morning, I peed on the stick, carried it upstairs and handed it to Nick. He was on the bed with Jett watching something on the computer. Jett was bouncing around. I was in my jammies so I started getting dressed for the day. Nick looked at the stick sadly. He asked Jett, "Hey, Jett, do you want a brother or a sister?" Jett stopped bouncing long enough to answer: "Yes."

"Well, you're gonna get one," Nick said. I looked up. Nick smiled mischievously at me and looked at the stick. "We're pregnant!" he announced. I screamed. I jumped up and down on the floor then on the bed. Jett looked scared. He never saw me act like that before. I kissed him all over and told him not to be scared, that mommy was very happy. Then he was happy too. We shared a family sandwich super hug. One little freakin' blue line changes everything.

Bittersweet Body Battles

vessel

Firm, perky, round breasts. Slender hips. Hands soft, hair coiffed. Cellulite only on my thighs. Exercise at will. Sleep till two. Dance all night. Love, eat, pray each day. My body. My way. Nine months once brings changes all around. Nine months twice makes reality profound. Brains, bones, blood. Hair, hips, hands. My body. Baby's way. One, two children in my veins. Mixing memories of firmness. Stirring softness into roughness. Pink-purple marks stretching battle wounds.

Remembering Belly

I'd heard through the mom grapevine that my body would remember what it was like to be pregnant and slip into pregnancy with ease. My belly remembered right away. I started showing significantly when I was only three months along. I looked like I was actually five months pregnant if I compared my belly to how it looked the first time. It went the same with my boobs; they started swelling right away.

I liked that my belly was fuller earlier on. It meant I could let it all hang out right away. Being pregnant gave me the freedom to not worry about how my body looked. It was a free pass in terms of dealing with my bodily insecurities, which were plentiful. I was thrilled we were pregnant again and I was happy my body was showing early so the rest of the world would know too.

It had felt like forever for my belly to start showing when I was pregnant with Jett. Then it had felt like forever for it to *stop* growing. My belly was huge. Everyone thought I was carrying twins. It was impossible for me to not be extremely aware of my growing belly. I rubbed and talked to it all the time. I paid close attention to everything baby-related that was going on with my body.

When I was pregnant with Miller a different kind of attention was paid to my belly. We knew it would grow. We knew it would be beautiful. But it wasn't just about Nick and me. It was about Jett too. It became a family affair to watch and feel it grow. Nick, Jett and I rubbed it and we all talked to it. I'm glad my belly remembered right away because it made Jett see how my body was changing. He could see that my belly was getting bigger so it made it easier for him to believe us when we told him there was a baby in it.

Jett never questioned how the baby got there. He was two-and-a-half when I got pregnant, old enough to understand what a baby was and accept our definitions about pregnancy. He was an amazing big brother even when Miller was in my belly. He couldn't wait to meet her. None of us could!

You're An Eight

When I was at camp as a child, there was a song I sang that used the lyrics 'you're an eight' instead of 'urinate.' It was cute. What happened to my ability to 'you're an eight,' however, was not so cute. I couldn't hold my pee in during certain situations. I come from a family of pee-when-you-laughers. My grandma, my aunts and my mother all squirt a bit when they laugh really hard. The potential for weak bladder control is in my genes. Having said this, there has been an obvious change in my ability to hold in my pee since both children have been born.

Coughing. Jumping. Sneezing. Laughing. Getting up quickly. All of these actions bring a tinkle to my drawers. After each delivery, and well past the eight-week mark (those weeks after labour when your body is supposed to miraculously return to a state of not-in-pain, not-swollen normal), my ability to not pee when doing certain things never recovered. After Jett was born, it took at least a year for me to be able to jump up and down without a little bit of pee squirting out. Even then, I couldn't do it for long. In order to sneeze and not pee, I had to cross my legs and tighten my vagina.

Running got yucky. I ran a few races after Miller

was born. One race had a few hills in it. Running up was challenging enough, but running down caused a waterfall in my tights. By the time I crossed the finish line, I was soaked in pee from crotch to knees. I had to sit on my jacket to drive home so I didn't get pee on the seat.

I met with my OB/GYN about it because I was wondering if this was going to change or if I should start to mentally prepare for life-long incontinence. She explained to me that the muscles in my uterus loosened because of child bearing thus causing a lack of support to the tube connecting to my urethra. The tube used to rest on my uterus, and if I sneezed, for example, the muscle of the uterus would cradle the tube in support and it wouldn't let any urine squirt out. Since the uterus had been stretched from childbirth, the support was weak and the tube couldn't hold the pee in as well.

I had options. I could continue to wait and see if my uterus strengthened. Consistently exercising would help. There was a surgery I could have that would insert a little net-like device for added support under the tube that connects to my urethra. She suggested I wait and see if things got better on their own before I thought about surgery. That was what I chose to do. Wait and see. For added safety, I went back to using tissues to help catch escaped pee.

Fart Fests And Burp-a-thons

Nick and I each have our own bottle of Tums on our bedside tables. Heartburn returned with a vengeance with baby number two. It erupted the worst when I'd lie down in bed at the end of my day. I read in one of my pregnancy books that you should try not to eat or drink at least two to three hours before going to bed. Yeah, right. That never happened in my world. It was no wonder that heartburn kicked in as soon as I lay down and there was nowhere for all that acid to go but back up my throat. I chose Tums as my antacid of choice and I Tumm-ed it up as often as I needed. Heartburn happened all the time and got worse at the beginning and end of the pregnancy.

Acid filled my esophagus and gas filled everywhere else. I could burp like a drunken man at a Super Bowl party and win awards for the belches I produced. It was amazing. My burping was a lot of fun for the family when I was pregnant with Miller.

Jett got a kick out of mommy's loud explosive releases of air. I surprised myself with the loudness and length of my burps. We had some big laughs post-belching. Fruit gave me great burps, especially apples. If I drank a Diet Coke, the burps would be memorably long. We made it a family event – burping with pregnant mommy. It was sure to bring smiles all around. I just had to remember to say excuse me after.

I had definitely burped like a mad woman while I was pregnant with Jett. There had been so much happening in my belly and guts, I couldn't help but be a belching queen. If I were a boxer, I would be named Gaseous Clay and burp and fart my way to a title belt.

I had always enjoyed farting, and I liked to believe that I did it well. This ability didn't change when I was pregnant. In fact, it only got better. During both pregnancies I was a fart master. Only after Jett was born and my ulcerative colitis flared up did the farting stop. This was a bizarre side affect of the disease – no farting. Can you imagine not farting and feeling that warm release of stinky air? That's how it was while I was sick. But once I healed up and my guts got back to normal, the farts began again. Since I didn't get sick after Miller was born, my farting extravaganzas continued in full force. I told Nick that he wasn't allowed to get mad if I warned him a stinky fart was coming. I did my best to warn him when I was going to let one loose.

Broccoli, edamame beans, sausages, carrots, apples, garlic, pop; these things gave me gas. I always had to be aware of what I put in my mouth and how it affected my body. I had to be extra aware of this when I was breastfeeding because everything I ate went right to the baby. If it would give me gas, it was going to give the baby gas. I didn't know that my guts would become a gurgling, gaseous, hot, stinky fart zone when I ate that sausage for dinner. But they did. Then I breastfed Miller and we both spent the night farting up a smelly storm. Needless to say, I never ate sausages again while I was nursing!

Baby Got Back Pain

I wasn't expecting the lower back pain when it came during my second pregnancy. It started about four months in and got progressively worse. It was coming from a muscle near my sciatic nerve. Apparently, there was a muscle that wrapped around my sit bone (or sacrum). This muscle extended up into my buttocks and lower back and it freaked out because the arch of my lower back was overworked. I had a pretty arched lower back to begin with, and when I added a heavy belly to the situation, the muscles just couldn't handle it. They were compensating for the arch and trying to support my spine. My chiropractor straightened me out. He explained why I was feeling pain and did his best to massage it out. What a relief! I visited a chiropractor or a massage therapist once a week during my eighth month of pregnancy to help ease the pain.

I remember one afternoon while getting changed I ran my hands over my lower back. All the muscles running up the sides of my spine were swollen. My spine was tucked in a valley between two hills of inflamed muscles. If I had lain down on my belly, I could have put liquid in the valley and it would have stayed there.

If my back went into a subtle spasm, which it did every once and a while, I'd have to slowly bend and stretch it out. If it happened in bed during the night, I'd call for Nick and he would gently rub it out. I had some lower back pain when I was pregnant with Jett but nothing like the pain I had when I was expecting Miller. The pain with Miller was intense and constant.

Although my back hurt all the time, I didn't let it stop me. I still lifted laundry baskets, vacuum cleaners and Jett. I know lifting these things wasn't helping the situation, but what was I supposed to do? Not do laundry? I wish. Not vacuum the house? Still wishing here. Not carry Jett? Not a chance.

If A Cramp Happens Does Anybody Hear It?

When I was eight months pregnant, and my bladder was getting squished by a five pound (or more) growing baby, drinking lots of water was a challenge if I wasn't strapped to a toilet. Unfortunately, according to my aqua fitness teacher, my lack of drinking water was the cause of the painful leg cramps that were tearing up my calves.

I'd wake up in the middle of the night with a knot the size of a golf ball in my calve muscles. It was like someone was stabbing me in the leg and then squeezing the wound. I could barely reach down to massage it out because my belly was too big.

One night I was having trouble sleeping because Nick was snoring and I was sweating like mad. I went to the couch and after cooling off in snoreless bliss I finally fell asleep. It wasn't long before I was rudely awakened by a growing cramp in my calf. I reached down over my belly as best as I could to grab my muscle. I flexed and pointed my feet and screamed out in pain to no one and everyone. I hoped Nick would hear me and come downstairs to help. He didn't hear a sound. His snoring was louder. I managed to breathe through the pain and wait for the cramp to subside on its own. Then I laughed really hard to myself, at myself. I rubbed my belly, which I had no problem reaching at all, and thought, *that was brutal – freakin' brutal.*

The next morning, I asked Nick if he heard me screaming in pain. He said no, and told me I should have gone to get him. I asked him how I was supposed to walk up two flights of stairs with a cramp in my leg. "Very carefully" was his witty response. He told me, "I'm sorry it happened. Leg cramps suck." I agreed.

Eighth Wonder

I had expected my feet to swell while I was pregnant with Jett. In the summer months, the humidity and heat touched my feet like a magic wand and turned them into what looked like loaves of bread. Puffy, sticky, maybe stinky, potentially painful loaves of feet bread. It was a good thing I had shoes that allowed for easy removal and room for my feet to swell into or out of.

I had become the proud owner of cankles. You know, when there is no visual break between where your calves end and your feet begin.

I was nine months pregnant with Jett by the end of May. It was flip-flop season so when my feet did get puffy, it was noticeable but comfortable. Because I had Miller in the fall, my feet didn't swell that much. When I was traveling and had walked all day, my feet did get sore and swell a bit but nothing too drastic. Nothing like how they swelled after labour with Jett.

My feet had been so swollen two days after Jett was born that they had become the eighth wonder of our family's world. People came from across town to see my loaves of feet. I was told the reason they swelled to a grotesque size was because of the epidural. There was so much of it in my system, it had nowhere to go but down. It all ended up in my feet. Yes, it was the drugs that baked my poor little feet into thick, stubby, loafy nubs. They looked like elephant feet with red toenails. I took a picture. Of course I took a picture.

Bittersweet Body Battle

I knew what my body was in for when I got pregnant the second time. I knew I'd get a big belly, the cellulite would be back in full force and my boobs would turn into bowling balls. I knew I would have to push the baby out and it would hurt like a cuss word. Once again, I had to give my body over to the baby growing inside of me. The bliss of being pregnant the first time was long gone.

My relationship with my body during the second pregnancy was easier because I knew I could do it. I could be pregnant, go through labour, and survive those painfully magical eight weeks after. I wasn't waiting on and tallying every single thing my body felt, not only because I'd done it before, but because I just didn't have the time or energy to focus this much attention on my body. It was relieving to give in, embrace, and understand that being pregnant would turn my body into a vessel that I needed to nurture.

Although it absolutely was a different physical experience being pregnant again, I wasn't hanging on my body's every change. I went with the flow even when it was painful and I couldn't get up off the couch without help. In my mind I knew that when it was all done, my body would be mine again.

What was different the second time was that I wanted my body back. I hadn't felt that way the first time. I had been infatuated with everything about pregnancy, painful or not. Thinking about getting my body back hadn't been anywhere in my mind. After Jett was born, my body was in bad shape because of an ulcerative colitis flare up. My main focus had been to heal. By default my body lost the baby weight, and regained its strength. Losing weight and getting my strength back after Miller was born was a different story.

I felt guilty for wanting my body back because I was nursing. My boobs were Miller's for all intents and purposes. I watched what I ate and drank because what I put in my body was directly related to her. I couldn't rush getting my body back because it still wasn't mine to take. It was difficult. I had to be patient. As time passed, and energy returned to my body, I started exercising and the desire to stop nursing increased. I was constantly battling in my mind about what to do.

When I stopped nursing and truly had my body back it was bittersweet. I regained a strong physical connection with myself yet shifted away from the special bonding experience I felt while nursing.

During my pregnancy with Miller, my relationship with exercise was different than it was with Jett. I thought a lot about exercise. Yes, *thought* about it. I wanted to get outside and walk or run but I mostly didn't. I was too busy and too tired. There were a few times when I made the time to go for a walk or a swim. I got big quickly, which didn't make exercising any easier. I was working full-time making a film and raising a two-year-old in a house with two flights of stairs. Let's just say I got my exercise via everyday activities. Exercise was important, don't get me wrong. In my mind I knew this, but my body couldn't follow through.

I didn't feel fat or gross. I didn't gain as much weight as I had during the first pregnancy. The pressure I had put on myself the first time to avoid gaining weight and worrying about losing it after just wasn't there with Miller. I had exercised a lot during the first five months of pregnancy with Jett. I had the time and the energy. I didn't do this the second time around. I was too exhausted all the time. I ate a bit healthier, slept as much as I could and let my body do what it already knew how to do: be pregnant.

The Demon Woman

I have a demon woman in my head. I'm certain she's a direct descendant of the demon woman in my mother's head. She has a perfect body and she will do everything she can to convince me that I should have one too. Sometimes her body is like Pink's or Audrey Hepburn's. Other times it's like Jennifer Aniston's or Katie Holmes' (but shorter). On any given day, in any given moment, she stands atop my brain, hands on her hips, watching me, judging me. She holds the reins to my hunger. She tells me I'm starving then she chokes me with disgust as I put food in my mouth.

After Jett was born, by virtue of being sick with ulcerative colitis, and being unable to keep any food in my body, I dropped my post-baby weight like a baby drops her soother. I weighed 118 lbs, which is the minimum weight a person of my height and age should weigh. I was too thin and looked sick. I had lost my baby weight, but not in a natural or safe way.

I was as healthy as could be after Miller was born. No flare up in sight, so losing my post-baby weight would have to be done by watching what I ate and exercising. Breastfeeding helped. Miller successfully helped suck away some of the weight I'd gained. I weighed just over 150 lbs after she was born, and I wanted to get down to 135 lbs. This had been my weight for the majority of my life.

I tried to lose weight on my own by being aware of what I was eating and exercising as often as I could. It wasn't working. I ate healthy, but the weight wasn't coming off. I decided to join Weight Watchers. My sister was getting married so I had a goal date in terms of losing my first chunk of weight. My mom and aunt had done it in the past so I knew it worked. When I went online to check it out, they were having a sale. I determined it was meant to be and joined.

I realized that while I was eating good food, my portioning was off. I wasn't eating poorly, but I was eating too much. I liked the format of the Weight Watchers plan and dedicated myself to following the rules and making better food choices. This wasn't easy. The demon woman didn't give me a break when I joined Weight Watchers. Oh no, she held up a point card each time I put a piece of food near my mouth.

I will reveal a secret now. I have low self-esteem when it comes to my body image. For as long as I can remember, it has been this way. I've always been on some form of diet or exercising extremely hard so I could lose weight and have a better-looking body. A better-looking body according to whom? To the demon woman? To my low self-esteem? Nick tells me I'm beautiful every day. I'm not exaggerating here. At least once a day he tells me I'm beautiful and may even be specific about which part of me. For example, he'll say, "Baby, you've got a great ass." I hear his compliment, but I don't often feel it or agree.

I compare myself to Jennifer or Katie and think less of myself because my body doesn't look like theirs. It doesn't seem to matter to me that people probably cook meals for these women, drag them out of bed to exercise, and do all the planning and organizing it takes to have and maintain the bodies that they have.

The point is it shouldn't matter. I shouldn't compare myself to these women or any women. I should love the body I'm in. I should take care of it and nurture it with healthy food choices and exercise. *I should.*

The demon woman still resides in my brain. I should evict her or at least ignore her. This is difficult for me. Maybe one day I'll believe what Nick so lovingly tells me, that I am beautiful.

Leftovers

I call what remains of my baby belly 'leftovers.' My tummy is by no means flat. White, spiderweb-like stretch marks scatter around my belly button. I have three thick stretch marks that look like some sort of jungle cat scratched me on each hip and a few subtle stretch marks on my inner thighs. My boobs share the same marked fate.

I don't mind my stretch marks. They are what remain of two fantastic pregnancies, a permanent physical reminder of the journey my body went through to have kids. Sometimes I get a little self-conscious if my belly shows, but I would get embarrassed even before the stretch marks were there. I'd love to have a flat belly but don't think it's in my cards. It would be okay if the stretch marks were there and the jiggly belly-ness wasn't.

I told Jett I was trying to lose weight so my belly would get smaller. He asked me why. I didn't have a good answer. Then he told me that he loves my belly, and it's stuck to me anyway, so how was I gonna get it off? Man, kids are smart. I had a bit of a belly even before I had Jett. It came from a long line of bellies that reach far back into my family's genetic pool. After an exercise class one morning, my gym instructor asked me if I was pregnant.

I wasn't, but my belly looked like it. She was so embarrassed. I told her not to worry. Really. I often get stopped and asked when I'm due. I gently rub my belly, swallow my embarrassment and say, "I'm not, these are my leftovers."

Final Conceptions

choose this house

Sex is laying bricks. One by one place each beautifully flawed, rough, solid, strong square on top, beside another. Pregnancy is adding windows. Look inside. Open. Accept the breeze. Feel the change. Lay more bricks. Respect the foundation. Appreciate the challenge. Labour is attaching the roof. Climb a ladder. Reach that height. Hammer nail after nail after nail. Preserve your sanctuary. Let Nature take her course. Protect your dwelling. Family is a house. Brick by brick, windowed, roofed, love is birthed. Fear is the big, bad wolf. He can't blow your house down. Invite him in. Offer him cake.

Tell the truth in this house. Be vulnerable in this house. Choose this house. You dreamt it into reality. You loved it into being. Believe in this house. Sex is laying bricks. One by one, beautifully flawed, rough, solid, strong square.

The Cross It Off Tour

A pretty amazing phenomenon happened when I celebrated my 28th birthday. I was born on Sunday, May 28th, 1978. Jett was born on Sunday, May 28th, 2006, twenty-eight years later to the day. I had celebrated my champagne birthday by getting the best gift I could get – a child.

I turned thirty while I was pregnant with Miller. This was a momentous event for me. I wanted to do something fabulous and daring that I could do while I was six months pregnant. Skydiving, mountain climbing or anything physically challenging was out of the question.

I always wanted to sing a live concert. Could I sing? I could carry a tune. Could I play an instrument? I could strum a few chords. Had I ever sang live before? In a high school musical when I was fifteen, half my age and half my size. It was settled. A live concert was the perfect gift I could give myself.

I hired a sound person, chose a location, and rented chairs and all the musical gear that was needed. I put together a list of my favourite poignant, life-anthem songs, contacted a musician friend of mine and begged him to rekindle our high school connection and accompany me at my concert. He said yes!

We worked out a secret rehearsal schedule because I wanted the concert to be a surprise. The only person who knew was my mom because she would watch Jett while my friend came over and we rehearsed. I designed invitations and sent them to about thirty people (my family and closest friends). I even sent one to our house for Nick. No one knew what was happening. All they got was a postcard in the mail that said: *"The Cross It Off Tour – Turning Thirty is Cool." Please attend a special concert on this day at this time at this location.*

I called it "The Cross It Off Tour" because I planned on sharing stories from my life when I crossed things off my 'List of Things to Do Before I Die.' The songs I chose were directly related to these life-changing, list-crossing events. I put a small card and a pen on each chair so that, during the concert, people could write their own lists and maybe begin to cross items off theirs as well.

My birthday came. Family and close friends arrived at the location completely unaware of what they were about to experience. I decorated our work studio like a concert hall, had pop and chips, and fancy lighting. I was so nervous, but I couldn't let a little thing like nerves stop me. I sang twelve songs and opened with "Like a Virgin" by Madonna. She's my favourite musician and I knew it would be hysterical to see a fat pregnant woman dancing to a song about virgins.

People sang along to John Lennon's "Imagine." They cried when I sang "Feels Like Home" by Chantal Kreviazuk and dedicated it to Nick and we all laughed when I sang "Hit Me Baby One More Time" by Britney Spears. I strutted and gyrated. It was too funny. One of the guys from work set up a camera and videotaped the show. There was a brief intermission so we could mingle. Jett came too, although he was a little confused because I was singing and he couldn't understand why I wouldn't stop to play with him. It was one of the craziest and most invigorating things I ever did.

Spiritual Things

I loved being pregnant the first time and I loved it again the second time. Even though it was hard on my body, I loved having a huge belly busting out of my centre. I liked the way my body looked in most outfits and for the second time in my life, I wasn't shy of my belly. I wanted to make sure that I did some special things for myself while I was pregnant. Spiritual things.

When I was pregnant with Jett, I asked the most spiritual woman I knew if there was anything she could suggest I do with my girlfriends to celebrate being pregnant. She said there was a Navajo ritual called a Blessing Way that celebrated a woman's transition into motherhood. This friend had become a Shaman (a medium between the visible world and the spirit world) and she said she'd be honoured to lead the ritual. The tradition called for a time when the women closest to me could gather together, sit in a circle, celebrate being women, and sing and bless my pregnancy and labour.

She told me to choose a date and a place and leave the rest to her. I had no idea what was going to happen on the day. I chose my house as the location, and told Nick he had to be somewhere else for the day. I left so they could set up. When I got back, I saw that the living room had been decorated with fresh flowers and it smelled like a forest of essential oils. The room had been transformed into a feminine palace. Each woman had a role to play from cooking to reading to massaging my feet and hands. We talked about how we knew each other and how each woman related to my life. I got to know everyone on a deeper level; I was filled with so much love.

My sister couldn't come because she had strep throat. I didn't want to catch it so I had to tell her that she and I would do something special just the two of us. On a Saturday we were both free, we drove to a beach in the county. We wrote in our journals, ate junk food, talked about life and love. We took pictures and dreamt out loud about what it would be like for her to be an aunt and for me to be a mother.

I wanted to do something similar when I was pregnant the second time, but on a smaller scale. I planned a special Blessing Way with my mom and my sister at my mom's house. We ate, danced, drew, laughed and took pictures. We put together a sacred altar that included a few special things from each of our lives. I brought some stones my deceased grandmother had given me, photos of Nick and Jett, a piece of chocolate and a photo of my dad. My sister is an artist, so she led us in a drawing exercise about what we envisioned the baby's spirit to be. We each created a beautiful piece of artwork. My mom told us stories about when she was pregnant with each of us.

Being pregnant had my creative juices flowing and

I did what I could to let them out. I had a friend of mine paint a bread bun in an oven on my belly when I was pregnant with Jett. We sat on the back porch of her house on a hot sunny day and talked about art and being moms. I took one of my sister's art classes and did a paper maché of my belly. Each creative experience I had among my female friends and family was a blessing in every way.

Neither Tom Nor Cruise

Late one night, Nick and I were in bed watching a film called *That's Entertainment!* We watched Bing Crosby and Gene Kelly sing and dance. Judy Garland, Jean Harlowe, Fred Astaire, Ginger Rogers – all the greats were there, swayin' and swaggerin'. Then this leggy brunette danced herself on screen. She sang beautifully. Her name was Ann Miller. Nick and I looked at each other and at the same time said, "Miller." We were nine months pregnant and we hadn't decided on a name yet. I told Nick that if we remembered the name in the morning, then we would choose it for baby number two.

The next morning, we awoke, looked at each other and said, "Miller it is." That's how we chose Miller's name. We knew it would suit a girl or a boy. Up to that point, we didn't talk much about names. We had a few flying around, but the only other name that was sticking was Tate. We liked Sophia, but everywhere we went people were naming their girls Sophia. We wanted our name to be different. Jett wanted to name the baby Superman. We were very relieved when we told him we'd be naming the baby Miller, and he gave us his approval.

What was crazy was that while we were pregnant,

Nick wrote a script for a feature film and the main character's name was Daniel Miller. Yup. Miller. This was the film we were working on while I was pregnant. We shot the film until September 27th, 2008. I gave birth to Miller on September 30th. Not once did we make the name connection.

What to name our first-born had been a big deal. We had talked about it a lot and we agreed that we wanted a name that was unique yet meaningful. We were filmmakers by trade and we just adored movies. Nick had always loved the name Jett. It was the name of the character that James Dean played in his last film, *Giant*. My favourite actor then – and now – was Tom Cruise. Neither Tom nor Cruise made the list. I had liked the name Jett a lot, and it would work for either a boy or a girl. It had been important to me that I knew well in advance what we'd name our child. It was on my 'list of things to do while pregnant.' With baby number two, the need to know wasn't as important. I knew a name would come. It did and we loved it.

Tearing Off The Layers

We asked Jett if he wanted a sibling. He said, yes, a sister. We told him we'd do our best to make one. At every step of the pregnancy, we kept him in the loop. He was there when the blue line showed up on the pregnancy test and I ran around the bedroom screaming in happiness. He was there as my belly grew. We touched it and talked to it together. We sang and read to it. He felt the baby kick and stared at me in awe.

He was never negative about the situation. Most of the time, we kept our schedule as consistent as possible. As we put the nursery together, and started getting out the baby clothes and toys and buying diapers, he noticed the changes, but we kept his life busy and normal.

Jett was in the early stages of toilet training. All the books said it would be difficult to start anything big like toilet training when a new sibling was on the way or newly arrived, but we still wanted to pursue it. He was doing well with it so we just went with the flow. He liked wearing Pull-Ups and sitting on the potty in his bedroom. Our goal was to have him toilet trained by the time the baby came. We didn't want to have to pay for double the diapers. He wasn't trained by the time Miller was born, but he mastered it soon after.

While I was pregnant with Miller, I was watching an entertainment show and someone was interviewing Angelina Jolie. They were asking her about being a parent and how she and Brad dealt with bringing a new baby home. I listened attentively to her answer. She said they had the kids prepare a welcome home party for the new baby, complete with decorations, cake and presents. This way, it gave the kids something to do while mommy and daddy were at the hospital and it made them feel like part of the situation. She said they also had gifts from the new baby for the existing kids.

Her advice, whether she realized she was giving it or not, was brilliant. I told Nick about it and we agreed it would be perfect to get Jett involved in a welcome home party for Miller. We included our parents and family members in the party too as they would be the ones preparing it while we were at the hospital in labour. Jett was thrilled about the whole idea. He and I shopped for the party beforehand. He picked out a gift for the baby, which he was convinced was a girl.

I went into labour for Miller very early on a Tuesday morning. My mom came over so she could be with Jett while we were at the hospital. He didn't see us leave in the morning, but we made sure that we kissed him goodbye. When he woke up, my mom told him that the new baby was coming. She was able to bring Jett to daycare that morning, and then pick him up later that afternoon. We did our best to keep his day as unaffected as possible.

After my mom brought Jett to daycare, she joined us in the delivery room and was there when Miller was born. It was a miraculous event that we were thrilled she was present for. She cried the whole time. When Jett was born, only Nick and I were in the delivery room. We wanted it that way. I'm glad we made that decision. Miller's labour was much easier, and because we knew what we could potentially be in for (we had been in labour for twenty-seven hours with Jett!) it was okay for us if my mom was there. Plus, I knew how happy it would make her to join us. We're grateful she was there.

People warned us that Jett would get jealous, angry and possessive when the new baby came home. He was none of those things. He was full of joyful expectancy and excitement, which I believe was directly related to how Nick and I included him in every step of the pregnancy. Only once did he ask me if I could put Miller back in my belly. I told him nope, sorry. He shrugged his shoulders and accepted our new reality.

I felt unwrapped by the time Miller came home. In a good way. I felt like I learned to tear off the layers of worry and paranoia that I had wound so tightly around myself when Jett came home. Don't get me wrong, I wasn't being careless or unrealistic. I wasn't fearful or overly concerned. I just felt ready. Ready for the unexpected, which is the most prepared I could be as the mother of *two* children.

Am Pregnant – Will Travel

Sunday, June 15, 2008 - I'm sitting at a small, round table in the loft of an old farmhouse in Vitteaux, France. There is a large, square window in front of me. The view outside the window is dreamy. Rolling hills are covered in different kinds of harvested farms or in grass where fat, white cows graze and sleep. It looks like a quilt sewn together by the hands of heaven. Birds fly in and out of my window view, fluttering like hyper kids in a schoolyard at recess. I can't hear them, but I know they are talking to each other, planning, playing, working.

I arrived in Paris, France on Thursday. Traveled by car to Vitteaux on Saturday, and will remain here until next Monday.

So many books about writing begin with the writer telling me about some fantastic place they've traveled to in order to write the book I am reading. It seems like in order to get a great manuscript written one has to leave her ordinary life. Step, fly, bike, drive, train away from all that is 'normal.' And do this alone. Leave your partner, children, family, co-workers and all that is generally safe and busy, to write.

I was seven months pregnant with Miller when I traveled to the Burgundy region in France for a twelve-day creative writing retreat. The excerpt above was from an email I wrote when I arrived at the farm where the retreat was held.

I hadn't done any extensive traveling while I was pregnant with Jett. We had been too poor and I had been working full-time at a place where the hours were inconsistent. It had been too hard to go away within the confines of shift-work. That wasn't to say I didn't want to, but our situation was different. Everything from where we lived to how much money we had was extremely different. I hadn't yet figured out who I was going to be as a mother. The pregnancy with Jett was very much about preparing myself, my body, my mind for the transition into motherhood. Being pregnant the second time was a bit easier in this way. I'd been mothering for two years. I kind of knew what I was in for and what to expect in terms of labour. Getting away felt like more of a realistic possibility.

This retreat brought one of my biggest writing dreams to life. Fly to Paris, drive through the rolling hills of Burgundy to a farm in Vitteaux, and write, write, write. I had been asked to attend the previous summer, but Jett was too young so I chose not to go. I remember how excited I was when I was asked to go again the following summer. We weren't pregnant yet but we were trying. I told the retreat leader that I wouldn't go if I was too pregnant or if I'd just given birth.

For months before I confirmed my attendance, I called the leader and told him if we were pregnant or not. One time, I left a message on his answering machine saying, "Guess what? I'm not pregnant!" His wife retrieved the message. We had some explaining to do! Needless to say, we got pregnant, and I calculated I would be in my seventh month of pregnancy during the trip. I made sure my OB/GYN said it was okay to travel at that point in my pregnancy. She gave me the go ahead.

Jett turned two at the end of May 2008. I hadn't been away from him for longer than a day and this trip marked the longest I was away from Nick since before we were married. While I was in France, my pregnancy rolled into its eighth month.

It was a massive decision for me to go on this trip. Nick and I talked for hours about it. He supported my desire to go because he understood what an amazing experience it would be for me. The trip would go like this: the first two nights were spent in Paris, the next eight were spent on the farm in Vitteaux and the final two were spent in Paris again.

I was scared. I had general worries about what could go wrong when traveling: plane crashes, lost luggage, stolen purse, no money or passport, getting lost. Throw into the mix: all of the above, while being seven months pregnant and the potential of going into labour on the plane ride there, in a foreign country or on the plane ride back.

I was scared that the people I was traveling and living with wouldn't like me, that it would be awkward between us because I was pregnant, and at such a different stage in my life.

Mostly, I was scared of being away from Jett and

Nick. I was scared that in my absence they would realize they didn't need me and they didn't love me anymore. These were ridiculous fears, but ones that I felt very strongly. I kept these particular fears nestled in the pages of my journal. I didn't want to give them life in spoken words, but they were very real.

A small part of me looked forward to not having to be a mother or wife, to not have to make dinner, vacuum, or tidy up eight thousand times a day. I looked forward to having a whole bed to myself. Mostly, I liked the idea of not having to worry about anyone but myself. It had been so long since I did anything alone that some days I felt giddy with excitement at the prospect of having such freedom. But the excitement was fleeting because I knew being a mother and wife was as natural to me as being a writer. I was giving myself the chance to wear a different hat for twelve days and I hadn't done this in years.

There were two main reasons why I think I had the courage to go to France. One was that it was the first real writing gift I'd given myself: a tried-and-true writer's retreat. Much of what it means to be a writer means identifying yourself as such. I could embrace this part of my identity at this retreat. I wanted to go and learn, even if it meant leaving everything that was safe and comforting, even if it meant leaving the people I loved the most.

The other reason was that I wasn't really alone. I had this big, round belly full of life that was with me all the time. Every time the baby moved, I got more energy. The baby would be in France with me and we would have this experience together. The thought of showing her photos of me pregnant with her, walking in breathtaking historical buildings and reading poetry in Paris would one day be a very special event I could share with her. As well, it would be amazing when I took her back to the places we were together when she was in my belly.

There were only a couple of things that I couldn't do because I was pregnant. I was in one of the richest wine making locations in the world and I couldn't participate in any drinking. I didn't know much about wine, and I didn't love the taste, but not drinking it certainly put me on the outskirts of sharing the same experiences with the others. The day the group went to a winery, I stayed at the farmhouse and wrote and slept.

Which brings me to another thing that being pregnant affected – my physical energy. In my mind, I was raring to go. My body, on the other hand, mostly wanted to sit or sleep. We spent a good portion of the day traveling to small, beautiful towns and getting history lessons about where we were. By the time we got back to the farm, which some nights wasn't until after 7pm, I was exhausted and starving. Dinner was always served about an hour after we returned.

Instead of going on some of the excursions, I stayed on the farm and rested because my body couldn't do it. I wrote what I could, then gave in to my exhaustion. Naps were essential – in the van or in bed, I took them often. My growing, round belly led me everywhere. The other writers were really supportive and I often had someone's hand on my belly waiting to feel a kick.

I was emotional. I cried every day, on my own in the early morning or late at night when the rest of the house was asleep or out. I cried because the ache in my heart for Nick and Jett was painful. If I had weighed my heart while I was traveling, it would have been heavier than ever before. It felt like a thousand pounds – all deeply and fully missing my family.

I also cried because of where I was and what I was doing. I was living a dream I'd had since I was small – to travel and write every day. Living a dream is an emotional upheaval. I was writing like never before. We had to read something after dinner each night, whether we wrote it or not. I always opted for the 'I wrote it' choice. It was scary, it made me vulnerable and sometimes I couldn't finish reading my poetry because I was crying so hard.

Thursday, June 19, 2008 – 7:05pm
The pain of realizing a dream is as strong as it takes to imagine it. This is really happening…from my head to my toes unbelievable. All I can do is cry.

At the end of the trip on the first night in Paris, we had the opportunity to read at the oldest bookstore in France, Shakespeare & Co. It was a three-level bookstore on the collar of the Seine in the floating shadows of Notre Dame. Its legacy stretched back to the fifties when writers like Hemingway and Fitzgerald, and artists like Picasso hung out there. Shakespeare & Co. was an artist's mecca, and I was there, pregnant and reading poetry that I'd penned.

Experiencing this reading was an extremely emotional event for me. Not only did it climax as the most amazing writing experience I'd ever had but it also meant that the trip was almost over. I could go home. After the reading, I went to a small café with two writers. There was a payphone nearby that I used to call home. When I heard Nick's voice, I broke down. I sobbed into the dirty handset wishing I were home. I would fly home the next afternoon, and it couldn't come fast enough. I could barely breathe. I sniffled and snotted all over the place. I talked briefly to Jett, barely holding off my tears so he wouldn't know I was freaking out. I didn't want to say goodbye.

I took a deep breath. The deepest I could muster at that point. I wiped my face and walked back to the café and the small, round table where we were sitting. I took one look at my writer friends. One had a family waiting for him at home too and I lost it again. My eyes exploded with tears, my nose with runny snot. My friend did his best to console me, hugging me as much as my giant belly would allow. I finally stopped crying. My tears left in their wake a puffy, red nose, swollen, pink eyes and shivering post-hard-cry hiccup sobs.

I kept to myself that night and the next day until we went to the airport and boarded the plane to fly home. I wanted to be quiet. To *feel* quiet and reflect on what I had done, how I had done it. I didn't write while I was on the plane, I read and slept. I thought I would write, but I couldn't. My focus was on getting home and seeing my family. Reading and sleeping made the time feel like it went by faster so that's what I did. I also knew I wouldn't be able to sleep at the whim of my body again when I got home. I took one last advantage of my sleep-when-I-want freedom.

Walking through the gate at the Windsor airport and seeing Jett run up to me was surreal. As a writer, I was different inside, but I had to leave my writer hat in my carry-on and don my mom and wife hats again. I did. With pride and gushing love.

Traveling to France was a unique opportunity I seized for my creative self. It made me a better mom because I realized that I *could* be all the parts of who I was – mother, wife, lover, writer, producer, swimmer, runner, daughter, sister, and on and on – and strive every day to find the balance to fit it all in. Being pregnant again gave me legs. Balancing legs. And I like to think I used them pretty well.

Acknowledgements

I have been pregnant for over two years and in labour for eight months with the child that is this book. There's no way I could have successfully managed its birth without the guidance, support and unconditional love from the following:

Father Quentin Johnson who I promised I'd dedicate my first book to. Thank you for your grace.

Janine Morris and Anne-Marie Charron, the first midwives to arrive on the scene and gently coax me through the beginning pains of contractions. Jane Christmas, my wise epidural who never wavered in her peaceful, painless support. Mary Ann Mulhern, John B Lee and Marilyn Gear Pilling, my pillows of inspiration and kindness.

Cameron Hucker, my 'other' boss who I can't thank enough for his patience. The Hargreaves, Kate and Paul (no relation!) for their grammar medicine. Mitch Albom, from across the river, for his passion for words that always keeps me pushing.

For Toni and Mo, the mothers whose strength and dedication I strive to emulate. Christopher Lawrence Menard, the match that lights my writing fire over and over again. My mother 'who borned me' in so many magical ways, and my sister who continues to be born. Mammy and D, my mattress princesses! The rest of my family and friends who helped give me time to write and cultivate this dream.

Miss Alice and Miss Laura, baby-watchers extraordinaire, who helped me breathe. For Dr. Suga, for taking care of my girl.

My medical editing team that held this baby in their arms and hearts and made sure she was perfect: Meghan Scanlan, Stewart McGowan, A.J. Nogeuira, Caitlin Lee, Brianne O'Grady, Samantha Murphy; Susie Heinrichs, Elizabeth Dyck, Krysta Fazio, Anna Hillner, Makenzie Morris, Lee Bagley. Jessica Minervini, whose guts are like mine – strong. Greg Pazuik, who wiped my tears and gave me my money suit. Dr. Marty Gervais, the best doctor in the business, who provided the safe space and unwavering love this baby needed to arrive (not only for baby, but for mommy too).

For Gooser, our first, who continues to inspire us all and make our hearts sing. Never stop inventing, Goose. I'll always be there for the build.

For Meeper, our second, who was with me when I got knocked up with this baby book. Meeps, you give me courage forever and for always. You're my girl.

And for Nick, my umbilical cord that connects me to everything I need. For his hot body and perfect penis. For the laughter we share and the tears too. I couldn't and wouldn't have birthed this book without you. Thank you. 'As you wish', baby. I love you.

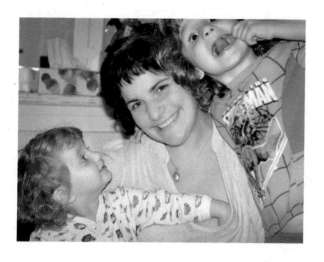

Born and raised in Windsor, Ontario, Vanessa Shields is an award-winning freelance writer whose work has been featured in both local and national publications. When she's not chasing after her two children with her husband Nick, she produces movies, writes poetry, and teaches creative writing.

"Vanessa Shields hold nothing back with her vivid, sometimes humorous, boldly honest account of her second pregnancy! She lays it all out, boobs, vagina, smells, discharges, sex, then and now! This book is a must-read for every woman, pregnant or not!"

Mary Ann Mulhern

"I love this book. Vanessa Shields has gone so deeply and honestly into her own experience that she has written a memoir that is universal in its relevance. The book is both a praise-song to the female body, and a wise and deeply moving testament to living with an open heart. I hope it ends up in the hands of every pregnant couple in North America."

Marilyn Gear Pilling

"I think there needs to be a balance of pregnancy books. Some of them seem so overwhelming and scary – all the things that can go wrong. Where are the books that talk about all the fun things that happen?"

Anonymous 26 year old Mother